CONTE

MIND-BODY RESET

A 30-DAY PROGRAM FOR BREAKING FREE FROM FOOD ADDICTION

BY STEPHANY DAVIS

Chapter 1. Unlocking Your Mind-Body Reset Journey

Hey there, fellow traveler on the road to wellness! Welcome to "Mind-Body Reset: A 30-Day Program for Breaking Free from Food Addiction." I'm thrilled you've picked up this book, because it tells me you're ready to embark on a transformative journey toward a healthier, more balanced life. So, grab a cozy blanket, a cup of tea, and let's dive into a conversation about breaking free from the chains of food addiction.

The Food Addiction Puzzle

We live in a world where food is not just sustenance; it's an experience, a comfort, and sometimes, a companion. But what happens when that relationship with food becomes a little too cozy? When the late-night snacks turn into a routine and the emotional connection with food starts overshadowing the nutritional one?

That's where the concept of food addiction comes into play. It's not about demonizing food or promoting unrealistic ideals. No, it's about understanding the intricate dance between our minds and bodies and how food can become a crutch in that dance. We're not here to shame or blame; we're here to untangle the web and set you on a path to a healthier, happier you.

Why This Program?

You might be wondering, "Why a 30-day program?" Well, the answer is simple. Research suggests that it takes about 21 days to form a habit, and an additional 9 days can solidify that habit into a lasting lifestyle change. This 30-day journey is crafted not as a quick fix, but as a holistic program to rewire your mind, reset your habits, and revive your relationship with food.

But let's be real for a moment – change is hard. Breaking free from the chains of food addiction is a challenge, but it's a challenge worth taking. The next 30 days won't be about deprivation or extreme measures. Instead, it's an opportunity to rediscover the joy of eating, to understand the whispers of your body, and to cultivate a deep, lasting respect for the vessel that carries you through this beautiful journey called life.

What Lies Ahead

In the pages that follow, we'll unravel the layers of food addiction together. We'll explore the science behind it, peek into the emotional corners where it often lurks, and lay the groundwork for a healthier, more balanced existence. This isn't a one-size-fits-all approach. Instead, it's a toolkit filled with strategies, wisdom, and a dash of humor to help you tailor this program to your unique self.

This book isn't about extremes. It's about finding your equilibrium, that sweet spot where health and happiness intertwine. You won't be asked to give up your favorite foods forever or spend hours at the gym if that's not your jam. Instead, we'll focus on understanding the triggers, building new habits, and, most importantly, fostering self-compassion.

Your Mind-Body Connection

Before we dive into the nitty-gritty of the program, let's talk about the mind-body connection – the heartbeat of this journey. Your mind and body are not two separate entities; they're dance partners in this grand ballet of existence. Understanding how they influence each other is key to breaking free from food addiction.

Have you ever noticed how stress can lead to that late-night rendezvous with a bag of chips? Or how a nourishing meal can uplift your spirits on a gloomy day? That's the mind-body connection at work. We'll explore how your thoughts, emotions, and physical well-being are intertwined, and how nurturing this connection can be a game-changer in your relationship with food.

Your Journey, Your Pace

This book is your guide, but remember, you're the protagonist of this story. Your journey will be as unique as your fingerprint, and that's something to celebrate. The program is structured, but flexibility is its backbone. Life is unpredictable, and this journey is about learning to navigate those twists and turns without losing sight of your destination.

Feel free to linger on a page if it resonates with you, or skip ahead if you're eager to explore what's next. This isn't a race; it's a stroll through the garden of self-discovery. And just like any good garden, there will be moments of bloom and moments of rest. Embrace them all.

What's in Store

In the chapters ahead, we'll delve into the science behind food addiction, helping you understand the physiological and psychological elements at play. We'll identify your personal triggers and patterns, offering reflective exercises and journaling prompts to illuminate the path forward.

Nutrition and meal planning will take center stage as we explore the art of nourishing your body without sacrificing pleasure. We'll introduce you to the concept of mindful eating – a practice that goes beyond the plate, inviting you to savor every moment.

Breaking old habits and cultivating new ones is a core theme. We'll discuss strategies for overcoming cravings, introduce positive rituals, and guide you in building a support system that elevates your journey.

Emotional intelligence will become your ally as we explore the depths of understanding your emotions and adopting healthier coping mechanisms. We'll touch on the profound impact of stress, sleep, and exercise on your relationship with food and provide practical tips to integrate these elements into your daily life.

Each week will bring new insights and challenges, building upon the last. It's a crescendo towards a symphony of change, and you're holding the conductor's baton.

Let the Journey Begin

So, are you ready? Ready to unearth the patterns, redefine your relationship with food, and embrace a healthier, more vibrant version of yourself? If your heart whispered a "yes," then let the Mind-Body Reset journey begin.

Turn the page, and let's embark on this adventure together. The next 30 days are yours – a canvas waiting for the brushstrokes of your transformation. Let's paint a masterpiece.

CHAPTER 2. UNDERSTANDING FOOD ADDICTION: UNRAVELING THE PUZZLE

Hey there, fellow explorer! As we dive into the second chapter of our Mind-Body Reset journey, we're putting on our detective hats to unravel the mystery of food addiction. Picture this as a cozy investigation into the intricate workings of our minds and bodies. So, grab a comfy seat, maybe a pen and paper for notes, and let's embark on this enlightening adventure together.

The Psychological and Physiological Factors

Food addiction isn't a simple puzzle with just one piece. It's more like a complex jigsaw, where both psychological and physiological factors interlock to create a unique picture for each of us. So, let's peel back the layers.

Role of Neurotransmitters and Brain Chemistry: The Brain's Delicate Dance

Our brains are magnificent orchestrators of our daily symphony, and when it comes to food addiction, they play a crucial role. Neurotransmitters, those little messengers in our brain, are like the conductors of this symphony. Dopamine, serotonin, and other brain chemicals are the key players influencing our mood, pleasure, and reward systems.

When we eat something delicious, dopamine is released, creating a sense of pleasure and satisfaction. It's a beautiful dance, a harmonious melody of flavors and sensations. However, in the case of food addiction, this dance can become a little too intense. Over time, our brains might start craving more, seeking that pleasurable sensation as a way to cope with stress, boredom, or even as a reward for a tough day.

Understanding this dance, this delicate interplay of neurotransmitters, is the first step in regaining control. It's about recognizing when the music is playing too loud and learning how to find the right rhythm.

Emotional Triggers and Coping Mechanisms: Comfort Food and Beyond

Ever noticed how a pint of ice cream can seem like a warm hug on a tough day? Emotional triggers and coping mechanisms are like the supporting actors in our food addiction drama. They often sneak in when we least expect it, influencing our food choices and eating habits.

Stress, anxiety, loneliness – these emotions can act as powerful triggers, driving us toward certain foods for comfort. It's not just about satisfying hunger; it's about finding solace in the familiar taste of a favorite dish. Over time, this connection between emotions and food can become a well-worn path, leading us to reach for that bag of chips before we even realize it.

But fear not! Awareness is our secret weapon. By understanding these emotional triggers and the coping mechanisms we've developed, we can start to untangle the knot. Through self-reflection exercises and journaling, we'll shine a light on those moments when emotions take the lead, empowering you to reclaim control.

Identifying Personal Triggers and Patterns

Now that we've laid the groundwork, it's time to dive a little deeper into the specifics of your journey.

Remember, this is not a one-size-fits-all approach. We're all unique beings, and our triggers and patterns are as individual as our fingerprints.

Self-Reflection Exercises: The Mirror of Awareness

Imagine self-reflection as a mirror, reflecting the inner workings of your mind and heart. Through a series of exercises, we'll gently guide you to explore your relationship with food. What are the situations that lead to overeating? When do you find yourself reaching for that extra serving or the sugary snacks?

By answering these questions with honesty and kindness, you're peeling away the layers of habit to reveal the core patterns that may contribute to food addiction. It's not about judgment but about understanding, about becoming the compassionate observer of your own behaviors.

Journaling Prompts: Putting Pen to Paper

Ah, the power of the written word! Journaling is a fantastic tool for self-discovery. We'll provide prompts that encourage you to jot down your thoughts, feelings, and experiences. Consider your journal a safe space, free from judgment, where you can express yourself openly.

By putting pen to paper, you're not only externalizing your thoughts but also creating a tangible record of your journey. As you revisit these entries, you'll witness the evolution of your relationship with food and gain insights that might have eluded you in the hustle and bustle of daily life.

The Dance of Understanding

So, here we are, swaying to the rhythm of understanding food addiction. It's not just about knowing the science or identifying triggers; it's about embracing the dance, acknowledging the steps that led us here, and preparing to choreograph new ones.

As you engage with the self-reflection exercises and journaling prompts, remember that this is your personal exploration. There's no rush; take your time, savor the insights, and be kind to yourself. This is a journey, not a destination.

The Mind-Body Connection

With our detective hats firmly in place, let's segue into the next chapter – the captivating world of the mind-body connection. Get ready to explore how your thoughts, emotions, and physical well-being engage in a beautiful dance, and how nurturing this connection is key to breaking free from food addiction. Exciting, isn't it? Let's keep this adventure rolling!

CHAPTER 3. THE MIND-BODY CONNECTION: HARMONY IN THE SYMPHONY OF WELL-BEING

Welcome back, my fellow explorers, to the vibrant pages of "Mind-Body Reset." Today, our compass points us toward a realm of profound significance – the Mind-Body Connection. It's like discovering the secret language that your thoughts, emotions, and physical self-share, creating a symphony that orchestrates the grand ballet of your existence. So, put on your dancing shoes, and let's twirl into the heart of this captivating journey.

Exploration of the Interconnectedness

Imagine your mind and body as dance partners, swirling gracefully on the ballroom floor. The Mind-Body Connection is the intricate choreography that allows them to move seamlessly together. It's not just about what you think or what you feel; it's about how those thoughts and emotions waltz hand in hand with your physical well-being.

The Impact of Thoughts on the Body: Power of Positivity

Ever heard the phrase "mind over matter"? Well, there's truth in those words. Positive thoughts have a remarkable impact on your physical state. When you embrace an optimistic outlook, your body responds with a symphony of feel-good hormones, promoting overall well-being.

On the flip side, negative thoughts can cast a shadow on this dance. Stress, anxiety, and self-doubt can manifest physically, affecting everything from your sleep patterns to your digestion. Understanding this connection allows you to become the choreographer of your mental landscape, shaping it into a stage for positivity and resilience.

The Influence of Emotions on Physical Well-being: Embracing the Ebb and Flow

Emotions are the spice of life, adding flavor to our experiences. But just like in any good recipe, balance is key. Unchecked, intense emotions can create discord in the Mind-Body Connection.

For instance, stress triggers the release of cortisol, the infamous "stress hormone," affecting everything from your immune system to your metabolism. On the other hand, joy and laughter release endorphins, your body's natural mood lifters.

This isn't about suppressing emotions but about acknowledging their impact on your physical self. By recognizing the ebb and flow, you gain the power to navigate through life's emotional landscape with grace and resilience.

The Impact of Stress, Sleep, and Exercise on Food Addiction

Now that we've dipped our toes into the dance floor of the Mind-Body Connection, let's explore three key elements that can either lead this dance to bliss or trip it up: Stress, Sleep, and Exercise.

Stress: The Uninvited Guest

Stress, that unwelcome guest at the party of life, can significantly influence your relationship with food. It's not uncommon to find solace in the familiar taste of comfort foods when stress comes knocking. Why? Because these foods often trigger the release of serotonin, providing a momentary escape from the chaos.

Understanding this connection is crucial. It's not about eliminating stress (let's face it, life happens), but about finding healthier coping mechanisms. Through mindfulness and stress-management techniques, we'll equip you with tools to tame the stress dragon and prevent it from hijacking your Mind-Body Connection.

Sleep: The Restful Interlude

Ah, the sweet embrace of a good night's sleep! It's not just a reset button for your mind; it's a vital player in the Mind-Body Connection drama. Sleep deprivation can disrupt the delicate dance, affecting hormones that regulate appetite and increasing cravings for high-calorie, sugary snacks.

In our 24/7 world, sleep often takes a backseat. But fear not! We'll delve into the importance of quality sleep and offer practical tips to create a sleep sanctuary that nurtures both your mind and body.

Exercise: The Energetic Flourish

Cue the energetic flourish – it's time for exercise to take center stage! Physical activity is more than a means to sculpt your body; it's a catalyst for a harmonious Mind-Body Connection. Exercise releases endorphins, reduces stress, and improves sleep – a triple treat for breaking free from food addiction.

But here's the catch: find an exercise routine that you enjoy. Whether it's a brisk walk, a dance class, or a session of yoga, the goal is to infuse joy into your movement. We're not chasing perfection; we're chasing the joy of movement, and in doing so, fostering a positive relationship between your body and mind.

Techniques for Cultivating Mindfulness and Self-awareness

Now that we've unraveled the threads of the Mind-Body Connection, it's time to weave in the tapestry of mindfulness and self-awareness. These are not just buzzwords but powerful tools that empower you to be present in the moment, to listen to the whispers of your body, and to cultivate a deep understanding of your inner landscape.

Mindfulness Practices: The Art of Being Present

Mindfulness is like a gentle breeze that clears the fog, allowing you to see and experience life in its full spectrum. Whether it's mindful eating, meditation, or simple breath awareness, these practices anchor you in the present moment.

We'll explore techniques to incorporate mindfulness into your daily routine, offering a sanctuary of stillness in the midst of life's hustle. By practicing mindfulness, you become the observer of your thoughts and emotions, creating space for conscious choices, especially in the realm of food.

Self-awareness: The Compass of Personal Growth

Self-awareness is your compass, guiding you through the landscapes of your desires, fears, and aspirations. It's about understanding your motivations, acknowledging your strengths and weaknesses, and embracing the journey of personal growth.

Through reflective exercises and journaling prompts, we'll nurture the seeds of self-awareness. It's not about reaching a destination of perfection; it's about embracing the beautiful messiness of being human and allowing that awareness to illuminate the path to a healthier, more balanced relationship with food.

The Dance Floor of Transformation

As we waltz through the chapters of the Mind-Body Connection, remember that this isn't a performance but a dance of transformation. The steps may be small or grand, and that's perfectly okay. It's about relishing the rhythm of your unique Mind-Body Connection, finding joy in each sway and twirl.

In our next adventure, we'll delve into the heart of nutrition and meal planning, exploring how to nourish your body without sacrificing the pleasure of eating. Get ready for a feast of insights and practical tips as we continue our journey toward breaking free from the chains of food addiction. Until then, keep dancing to the melody of your Mind-Body Connection – the symphony of your well-being.

Chapter 4. Nutrition and Meal Planning: Nourishing Your Body, Savoring Life's Feast

Hello, fellow travelers! Welcome to the heart of our Mind-Body Reset journey – Nutrition and Meal Planning. Picture this as a delicious feast where we savor the flavors of wholesome nourishment without sacrificing the joy of eating. Today, we're donning our chef hats and diving into the world of balanced nutrition, mindful eating, and creating a meal plan that's both satisfying and sustainable. So, grab a seat at the table, and let's embark on this culinary adventure together.

Balanced and Nourishing Food Choices: The Art of Eating Well

Let's kick off our culinary journey by exploring the art of balanced and nourishing food choices. This isn't about deprivation or counting calories; it's about savoring the abundance of nature and treating your body as the cherished guest at life's banquet.

Understanding Macronutrients: The Building Blocks of Energy

Macronutrients – the superheroes of nutrition! These include carbohydrates, proteins, and fats, each playing a crucial role in fueling your body. Carbs are your body's preferred source of energy, proteins repair and build tissues, and fats provide essential nutrients for brain health and overall well-being.

But here's the twist: it's not about demonizing any macronutrient but about finding the right balance. We'll explore how to incorporate a variety of sources, ensuring your plate is a colorful mosaic of nutrients.

Micronutrients: The Magic of Vitamins and Minerals

Think of micronutrients as the enchanting spices that elevate your culinary masterpiece. Vitamins and minerals are the unsung heroes, supporting everything from bone health to immune function. Embracing a diverse and colorful array of fruits and vegetables ensures you're receiving a symphony of these micronutrients.

We'll delve into the rainbow of possibilities, offering practical tips to make your plate a canvas of vibrant, nutrient-rich choices. It's not just about eating; it's about celebrating the diversity of flavors and textures that nature provides.

Developing a Healthy Relationship with Food: Beyond the Plate

Eating is not just a physical act; it's a multisensory experience that engages your mind, body, and soul. Developing a healthy relationship with food goes beyond the nutrients on your plate; it's about savoring the journey of nourishment.

Mindful Eating: Savoring Each Bite

Ever devoured a meal without truly tasting it? Welcome to the world of mindful eating, where each bite is a moment to be savored. We'll explore techniques to bring mindfulness to your meals, from appreciating the colors and textures to tuning in to your body's hunger and fullness cues.

By slowing down and being present, you'll not only enhance the enjoyment of your food but also foster a deeper connection with your body's signals. It's a practice that transforms eating from a routine into a celebration of nourishment.

Creating a Healthy Eating Environment: The Atmosphere Matters

Picture this: a candlelit dinner versus a hurried meal at your desk. The environment in which you eat plays a significant role in your relationship with food. We'll discuss the importance of creating a positive and relaxed atmosphere for meals, allowing you to fully engage with the experience.

From setting a beautiful table to minimizing distractions, these simple adjustments can turn your meals into moments of joy and connection. It's about making every meal a celebration of self-care.

Creating a Sustainable and Realistic Meal Plan: The Roadmap to Success

Now, let's roll up our sleeves and create a meal plan – not a rigid set of rules, but a flexible roadmap that guides you toward your health and wellness goals.

Assessing Your Nutritional Needs: Tailoring the Plan to You

We're all unique individuals with different nutritional needs. Whether you're a busy parent, a working professional, or a free spirit on the go, your meal plan should align with your lifestyle. We'll guide you through an assessment of your nutritional requirements, considering factors such as age, activity level, and health goals.

This personalized approach ensures that your meal plan isn't a generic template but a bespoke guide crafted just for you. It's not about restriction; it's about creating a sustainable and enjoyable way of nourishing your body.

Meal Prep and Batch Cooking: Effortless and Efficient

Let's debunk a myth: Healthy eating doesn't mean spending hours in the kitchen each day. Enter the world of meal prep and batch cooking, where a little effort goes a long way. We'll share time-saving tips and easy recipes that allow you to prepare meals in advance, ensuring that wholesome choices are readily available when hunger strikes.

Meal prep is not just about efficiency; it's a self-care ritual, a way of honoring your well-being. We'll guide you through the steps, making this process as enjoyable as the meals themselves.

Building Balanced Meals: The Plate Method

Ever heard of the plate method? It's a simple yet powerful tool to ensure that your meals are well-balanced and nourishing. We'll explore how to divide your plate into sections for proteins, carbohydrates, and vegetables, creating a visual guide that takes the guesswork out of balanced eating.

This approach isn't about restrictive portion control; it's about creating a satisfying and sustainable way of eating. You'll soon discover that balance is not only achievable but also delicious.

Tips for Mindful Eating: Bringing It All Together

As we tie a bow around our culinary adventure, let's distill the essence of mindful eating into practical tips that you can integrate into your daily life.

Listen to Your Body: The Wisdom Within

Your body is a wise guide, providing signals of hunger and fullness. Tune in to these cues, honoring your body's natural rhythm. It's not about external rules but about cultivating a relationship with your body based on trust and respect.

Savor Each Bite: The Pleasure Principle

Eating is meant to be pleasurable. Slow down, engage your senses, and savor the flavors. Whether it's the crunch of a fresh apple or the warmth of a comforting soup, let each bite be an experience. Pleasure and nourishment go hand in hand.

Minimize Distractions: A Mindful Atmosphere

Create a mindful eating environment by minimizing distractions. Turn off the TV, put away the phone, and focus on the act of eating. This simple shift transforms your meals from a routine task into a moment of self-care.

Express Gratitude: A Ritual of Thanks

Before you dive into your meal, take a moment to express gratitude. Whether it's for the hands that prepared the food, the journey it took to reach your plate, or the nourishment it provides, gratitude enhances the mindful eating experience.

Recipes and Meal Planning Templates: Your Culinary Toolkit

To enrich your culinary journey, we've prepared a collection of delicious and nutritious recipes, ranging from quick snacks to hearty meals. These recipes are not about restriction but about expanding your culinary repertoire with flavors that nourish both body and soul.

Additionally, meal planning templates will serve as your culinary toolkit, providing a canvas to sketch out your weekly meals. Feel free to adapt and customize these templates to suit your preferences and schedule. This isn't a rigid structure but a flexible guide that empowers you to make nourishing choices with ease.

The Culinary Symphony Continues

As we wrap up our exploration of Nutrition and Meal Planning, remember that this isn't a fleeting moment but the beginning of a culinary symphony that will accompany you on your Mind-Body Reset journey. The flavors of balanced nutrition, mindful eating, and personalized meal planning will weave together to create a harmonious dance of well-being.

In our next chapter, we'll venture into the realm of breaking habits and establishing new ones – a pivotal step in reshaping your relationship with food. Until then, savor the joy of nourishment and relish the journey of cultivating a healthy, vibrant you. Bon appétit!

CHAPTER 5. BREAKING HABITS AND ESTABLISHING NEW ONES: A DANCE OF TRANSFORMATION

Hey there, fellow champions of change! As we journey through the chapters of "Mind-Body Reset," we find ourselves at a crossroads – the intersection of breaking old habits and paving the way for new ones. Imagine this as a dance floor where the steps of transformation unfold, and the rhythm of your journey begins to sync with the beat of positive change. So, lace up your dancing shoes, and let's explore the art of breaking free from old habits while crafting the dance of a new, empowered you.

Recognizing and Addressing Unhealthy Habits: Shedding Light on Shadows

Before we leap into the realm of establishing new habits, it's crucial to cast a spotlight on the shadows – those old, familiar habits that may be holding you back. Habits, whether big or small, shape the tapestry of our daily lives. They are the autopilot settings that guide our actions, often without conscious thought.

Self-Reflection: The Mirror of Awareness

The journey begins with self-reflection, an introspective dance that invites you to observe your habits without judgment. What are the patterns that no longer serve you? Which habits leave you feeling drained or dissatisfied?

Through guided self-reflection exercises, we'll navigate this introspective terrain. It's not about blame or guilt but about shedding light on the shadows, understanding the roots of these habits, and acknowledging the space for transformation.

Setting Realistic Goals: The Blueprint for Change

Goals are the compass that guides your journey. But here's the secret sauce – they need to be realistic, attainable, and aligned with your values. We'll delve into the art of setting SMART goals – Specific, Measurable, Achievable, Relevant, and Time-bound.

By breaking down your larger goals into smaller, actionable steps, you create a roadmap for change. It's not about radical overhauls; it's about gradual, sustainable progress that allows you to celebrate each milestone along the way.

Strategies for Overcoming Cravings: The Cravings Conundrum

Cravings – those pesky whispers that beckon you toward the familiar comforts of old habits. Whether it's the afternoon chocolate fix or the late-night snack attack, cravings often stand as gatekeepers to change. Fear not, for we shall equip you with strategies to navigate this cravings conundrum.

Understanding Triggers: Cracking the Code

Cravings are often triggered by specific cues, be it stress, boredom, or environmental triggers. By identifying these triggers, you gain the upper hand in understanding the root causes of your cravings. We'll embark on a journey of self-discovery, unraveling the threads that weave the tapestry of your habits.

Substitution, Not Deprivation: A Toolbox of Alternatives

Deprivation is the arch-nemesis of sustainable change. Rather than focusing on what you can't have, let's shift the spotlight to what you can enjoy. We'll introduce a toolbox of alternatives – healthy snacks, mindful activities, and strategies to redirect your focus when cravings strike.

Mindful Eating: A Shield Against Mindless Cravings

Mindful eating, our trusty ally from the previous chapter, is a powerful shield against mindless cravings. By savoring each bite and tuning in to your body's hunger and fullness cues, you cultivate a mindful approach to eating. It's not just about what you eat but how you eat, transforming the act of nourishment into a conscious, intentional experience.

Introducing Positive Habits and Rituals: The Dance of Transformation

Now that we've bid farewell to the old habits, it's time to welcome the new stars onto the stage – positive habits and rituals. These are the dancers that will shape the choreography of your daily life, infusing it with energy, purpose, and joy.

Start Small, Dream Big: The Power of Micro-Habits

Change doesn't have to be grandiose; in fact, it often thrives in the realm of micro-habits. These are tiny, manageable actions that, when repeated consistently, create a ripple effect of change. We'll explore the magic of starting small, introducing micro-habits that align with your goals and values.

Building a Routine: Your Daily Choreography

Routines provide the scaffolding for your habits to thrive. We'll guide you in crafting a daily routine that accommodates your new habits seamlessly. Whether it's a morning ritual that sets a positive tone for the day or an evening routine that promotes relaxation, routines become the canvas upon which your dance of transformation unfolds.

Accountability Partners: The Dance Troupe of Change

Change is often more fun and sustainable when it's a shared experience. Enter accountability partners, your dance troupe of change. Whether it's a friend, family member, or a like-minded companion on this journey, having someone to share your goals and victories creates a supportive, motivating environment.

Building a Support System: The Pillars of Transformation

As you waltz through the intricate steps of change, having a support system acts as the sturdy pillars that hold up the dance floor. Building connections with like-minded individuals, whether in person or through virtual communities, provides a network of encouragement, shared experiences, and collective wisdom.

Community Engagement: Sharing the Journey

Engaging with a community of individuals on a similar path amplifies the transformative power of change. Whether it's joining a local fitness group, participating in online forums, or attending workshops, the collective energy of a community can uplift, inspire, and fuel your journey.

Professional Support: Your Dance Instructors

Sometimes, seeking the guidance of professionals can be the key to refining your dance moves. Nutritionists, therapists, and fitness trainers are like experienced dance instructors, providing personalized guidance and expertise. We'll explore how incorporating professional support can enhance your Mind-Body Reset journey.

Week-by-Week Program: From Reflection to Transformation

Now that we've laid the groundwork, let's embark on a week-by-week program that blends the art of breaking habits with the magic of establishing new ones.

Week 1-2: Awareness and Reflection

- Dive into self-reflection exercises, identifying patterns and triggers.

- Set realistic, actionable goals for the upcoming weeks.
- Begin experimenting with micro-habits aligned with your goals.

Week 3-4: Breaking Unhealthy Habits

- Introduce strategies to overcome cravings, identifying triggers and alternatives.
- Engage in mindful eating practices, savoring each meal consciously.
- Start substituting unhealthy habits with positive alternatives.

Week 5-6: Establishing New Habits

- Dive into the world of micro-habits, building routines that align with your goals.
- Share your goals and progress with your accountability partners or community.

- Introduce professional support if needed, such as consulting a nutritionist or therapist.

Week 7-8: Strengthening Support Systems
- Reflect on the impact of your support system on your journey.
- Engage more actively with your chosen community, sharing experiences and insights.
- Evaluate the effectiveness of your routines and make adjustments as needed.

Maintaining Progress and Long-Term Success: The Grand Finale

As our dance of transformation progresses, the grand finale is not the end but a celebration of sustained progress and long-term success. Here are strategies to ensure that the steps you've embraced become a lifelong dance.

Regular Reflection: The Dance Floor Check-In

- Schedule regular moments of reflection to assess your progress and reassess your goals.
- Celebrate victories, both big and small, and acknowledge the journey you've traveled.

Adapting and Evolving: The Dance of Flexibility
- Embrace the ebb and flow of life, recognizing that change is a constant companion.
- Be open to adapting your routines, habits, and goals as your circumstances evolve.

Mindful Living: The Dance of Conscious Choice
- Continue to practice mindfulness in all areas of your life, making conscious choices that align with your values.
- Extend the principles of mindful eating to mindful living, fostering a holistic approach to well-being.

Celebrate Your Journey: A Dance of Gratitude

As we conclude this chapter on breaking habits and establishing new ones, take a moment to celebrate your journey. The dance floor of transformation is a place of courage, resilience, and self-discovery. Every step, stumble, and twirl contributes to the masterpiece that is your life.

Celebrate not just the destination but the beauty of the journey itself. Express gratitude for the strength within you, the support around you, and the dance of transformation that continues to unfold.

Moving Forward: The Dance Continues

As we bid adieu to this chapter, remember that the dance of transformation is an ongoing, evolving journey. In the chapters to come, we'll explore the profound impact of emotional intelligence, stress management, sleep, and exercise on your relationship with food.

Until then, keep dancing to the rhythm of positive change, and let the music of your journey resonate with the joy of transformation. You've got this!

CHAPTER 6. EMOTIONAL INTELLIGENCE AND COPING STRATEGIES: NAVIGATING THE SYMPHONY OF FEELING

Hello, dear companions on the path of self-discovery! As we venture deeper into the realms of the "Mind-Body Reset," our compass now points toward the intricate dance of Emotional Intelligence and Coping Strategies. Imagine this as a symphony where the melodies of your emotions harmonize with the rhythm of coping mechanisms, creating a masterpiece that resonates with balance and well-being. So, let's embark on this emotional journey together, exploring the art of understanding, embracing, and navigating the rich tapestry of our feelings.

The Essence of Emotional Intelligence: The Conductor of Self-Discovery

Emotional Intelligence (EI) is like the conductor of our internal symphony. It involves recognizing, understanding, and managing our own emotions, as well as empathizing with the emotions of others. As we delve into this chapter, let's unfold the layers of emotional intelligence, discovering how it shapes our responses, choices, and overall well-being.

Self-Awareness: The Prelude to Emotional Intelligence

The journey begins with self-awareness, the prelude to emotional intelligence. It's about tuning in to your own emotional landscape, understanding the nuances of your feelings, and recognizing how they influence your thoughts and actions.

Self-awareness allows you to navigate the labyrinth of emotions with clarity. Through reflective exercises and mindful practices, we'll cultivate the art of being present with our emotions, fostering a deeper understanding of the symphony within.

Self-Regulation: The Art of Emotional Balance

Once you've tuned into your emotions, the next step is self-regulation – the art of maintaining emotional balance. It's not about suppressing emotions but about responding to them in a constructive manner. We'll explore techniques such as mindfulness, deep breathing, and positive self-talk to navigate the waves of emotions with grace.

Understanding the ebb and flow of emotions empowers you to make conscious choices, ensuring that you remain in the driver's seat of your emotional journey. It's a dance of resilience and adaptability.

The Dance of Empathy: Nurturing Connection

Empathy, the dance partner of emotional intelligence, invites us to step into the shoes of others and share in their emotional experience. It's a profound form of connection that enriches relationships and enhances our understanding of the human experience.

Empathetic Listening: The Dance of Presence

Empathetic listening is the heartbeat of empathy. It involves being fully present with others, offering a non-judgmental space for them to express their emotions. Through this dance of presence, we deepen our connections, fostering an environment where emotions are acknowledged and valued.

Cultivating Compassion: The Ripple Effect

Empathy extends beyond understanding to action – it evolves into compassion. Cultivating compassion involves not only recognizing the emotions of others but also taking steps to alleviate their suffering. It's a ripple effect that creates a harmonious dance of shared humanity.

Coping Strategies: The Dance Partners of Resilience

Life is a dance of highs and lows, and coping strategies are the trusted dance partners that guide us through the twists and turns. In this section, we'll explore a repertoire of coping strategies – tools that empower you to navigate challenges, reduce stress, and nurture your emotional well-being.

Mindfulness and Meditation: The Dance of Presence

Mindfulness and meditation are timeless dance forms that invite you to be fully present in the moment. By cultivating a state of awareness, you can observe your thoughts and emotions without attachment, fostering a sense of calm and clarity. We'll introduce practical mindfulness exercises and meditation techniques to weave into your daily routine.

Creative Expression: The Dance of Artistry

Creativity is a powerful outlet for emotions, offering a canvas for self-expression. Whether it's through art, writing, music, or dance, creative expression becomes a dance of artistry that allows you to channel your emotions into a tangible form. We'll explore how engaging in creative pursuits can be both therapeutic and liberating.

Physical Activity: The Dance of Vitality

Movement is a language of its own, and physical activity becomes a dance of vitality. Exercise releases endorphins, the body's natural mood lifters, and provides a healthy outlet for stress. Whether it's a brisk walk, a dance session, or yoga, we'll guide you in incorporating joyful movement into your routine.

Positive Affirmations: The Dance of Encouragement

Words have the power to shape our reality, and positive affirmations become the dance of encouragement. By incorporating uplifting and affirming statements into your daily routine, you can shift your mindset and nurture a positive internal dialogue. We'll provide a collection of affirmations to inspire and empower.

Social Connection: The Dance of Community

Human connection is a dance of shared experiences, offering support and understanding. Whether it's spending time with loved ones, joining clubs or groups, or connecting with like-minded individuals, fostering social connections becomes a vital coping strategy. We'll explore the significance of community in nurturing emotional well-being.

Emotional Resilience: The Dance of Bouncing Back

Resilience is the dance of bouncing back from life's challenges, and emotional resilience is a key component of our coping dance. It's about navigating adversity, adapting to change, and emerging stronger on the other side. We'll delve into the elements that contribute to emotional resilience and explore strategies to cultivate this dance of inner strength.

Acceptance and Adaptability: The Dance of Flow

Life is a river of constant change, and acceptance is the dance of flowing with its currents. By embracing change and cultivating adaptability, you enhance your capacity to navigate challenges. We'll explore practices that foster acceptance and flexibility, empowering you to dance through the twists and turns of life.

Learning from Setbacks: The Dance of Growth

Setbacks are not the end but a pause in the dance, an opportunity for growth. By reframing challenges as lessons and learning experiences, you transform adversity into a dance of personal development. We'll guide you in navigating setbacks with resilience and using them as stepping stones toward a more empowered self.

Stress Management: The Dance of Harmony

Stress, the invisible partner in life's dance, requires a dance of harmony for balance and well-being. In this section, we'll explore stress management strategies that empower you to navigate the complexities of daily life with grace.

Time Management: The Dance of Balance

Time management is the dance of balance that ensures you have the space to prioritize self-care and reduce stress. We'll introduce practical techniques to manage your time effectively, allowing you to engage in activities that nurture your emotional well-being.

Mind-Body Techniques: The Dance of Integration

Mind and body are intertwined, and mind-body techniques become the dance of integration. Practices such as yoga, tai chi, and progressive muscle relaxation facilitate harmony between your mental and physical states. We'll guide you in incorporating these techniques into your routine for a holistic approach to stress management.

Developing Emotional Intelligence: A Personalized Program

Now that we've explored the components of emotional intelligence and coping strategies, let's craft a personalized program to enhance your emotional well-being. This program is a dance of self-discovery, designed to deepen your emotional intelligence and empower you with effective coping tools.

Week 1-2: Self-Reflection and Awareness

- Engage in daily journaling to reflect on your emotions and their triggers.
- Identify patterns in your emotional responses and reactions.
- Begin incorporating mindfulness exercises into your routine to enhance self-awareness.

Week 3-4: Empathy and Connection

- Practice empathetic listening in your interactions with others.
- Cultivate compassion by finding ways to support and connect with those around you.
- Join a community or group where you can share experiences and build connections.

Week 5-6: Coping Strategies Toolbox

- Experiment with different coping strategies, such as mindfulness, creative expression, and physical activity.
- Identify the strategies that resonate most with you and integrate them into your daily routine.

- Share your experiences with your support system, seeking feedback and encouragement.

Week 7-8: Emotional Resilience and Stress Management
- Explore the concept of acceptance and adaptability in the face of challenges.
- Embrace setbacks as opportunities for growth, reframing them as lessons.
- Develop a time management plan to create balance and reduce stress in your daily life.

The Ongoing Dance of Emotional Well-being

As we conclude this exploration of Emotional Intelligence and Coping Strategies, remember that this is not a one-time performance but an ongoing dance. Emotional well-being is a dynamic, evolving journey, and each step you take contributes to the symphony of your life.

Continue to practice self-awareness, nurture connections, and explore coping strategies that resonate with your unique dance. The chapters ahead will unravel the impact of sleep, exercise, and nutrition on your emotional well-being, offering a holistic approach to the Mind-Body Reset journey.

Until then, dance to the rhythm of your emotions, embracing each note as a unique expression of your beautiful, ever-evolving self. You're not alone on this dance floor – the symphony of your well-being continues to unfold. Dance on!

CHAPTER 7. EXERCISE AND MOVEMENT: THE JOYFUL DANCE OF WELL-BEING

Greetings, fellow enthusiasts of the Mind-Body Reset journey! As we step into the lively realm of Chapter VII, we find ourselves on the vibrant dance floor of Exercise and Movement. Imagine this as a joyful dance, a celebration of vitality, strength, and well-being. So, lace up your sneakers, let the music of motivation play, and let's groove together through the exhilarating world of physical activity.

The Rhythm of Exercise: A Symphony for Body and Mind

Exercise isn't just about breaking a sweat; it's a symphony that harmonizes your body and mind. In this section, we'll explore the multifaceted benefits of regular physical activity, understanding how it contributes to your overall well-being.

Physical Health: The Dance of Vitality

Exercise is the heartbeat of physical health, pumping life into every corner of your body. From cardiovascular fitness to improved muscle strength, the dance of vitality begins with movement. We'll unravel the physiological magic that occurs when you engage in regular exercise, enhancing your cardiovascular system, boosting metabolism, and promoting overall health.

Mental Well-Being: The Dance of Endorphins

Ever heard of the "runner's high"? It's not just a myth – it's the dance of endorphins, your body's natural mood lifters. Exercise has a profound impact on mental well-being, reducing stress, anxiety, and depression. We'll explore how the dance of endorphins can transform your mood, enhance cognitive function, and create a positive feedback loop for your brain.

Finding Your Dance: Exploring Different Forms of Exercise

The dance floor of exercise is vast and varied, offering a multitude of styles to suit every taste. Let's explore different forms of physical activity, helping you discover the dance that resonates most with your preferences and lifestyle.

Cardiovascular Exercise: The Dance of Stamina

Cardiovascular exercise, or cardio for short, is the dance of stamina that gets your heart pumping. Whether it's brisk walking, running, cycling, or dancing, cardio improves your cardiovascular health, increases endurance, and elevates your energy levels. We'll guide you in finding a cardio dance that aligns with your fitness goals and preferences.

Strength Training: The Dance of Resilience

Strength training is the dance of resilience, sculpting your muscles and fortifying your body. It involves lifting weights, using resistance bands, or practicing bodyweight exercises to build strength. We'll delve into the benefits of strength training, including improved metabolism, enhanced bone density, and a sculpted physique.

Flexibility and Mobility: The Dance of Grace

Flexibility and mobility are the dances of grace that enhance your range of motion and prevent stiffness. Yoga, Pilates, and stretching exercises contribute to flexibility, promoting joint health and reducing the risk of injury. We'll explore how incorporating these dances of grace into your routine enhances overall well-being.

Mind-Body Practices: The Dance of Harmony

Mind-body practices, such as yoga and tai chi, are the dances of harmony that unite physical movement with mindful awareness. These practices not only contribute to physical fitness but also foster mental calmness and stress reduction. We'll guide you through the serene movements of mind-body practices, helping you find a dance that nurtures both body and soul.

The Dance of Motivation: Cultivating a Love for Movement

Embarking on the dance of exercise requires a sprinkle of motivation – the magical ingredient that transforms movement from a chore into a joyful ritual.

Let's explore strategies to cultivate and sustain motivation, ensuring that your dance with exercise becomes a lifelong journey.

Setting Realistic Goals: The Dance of Progress

Goals are the stepping stones that guide your dance of progress. By setting realistic, achievable goals, you create a roadmap for success. We'll delve into the art of goal-setting, ensuring that your aspirations are motivating, measurable, and aligned with your overall well-being.

Variety and Fun: The Dance of Enjoyment

Exercise shouldn't be a monotonous routine but a dance of enjoyment that brings a smile to your face. Incorporating variety into your routine, trying new activities, and embracing the fun side of movement make the dance of exercise an exciting adventure. We'll explore ways to infuse enjoyment into your routine, making it a highlight of your day.

Accountability Partners: The Dance Troupe of Support

A dance is often more enjoyable when shared with others. Accountability partners, whether friends, family, or workout buddies, become your dance troupe of support. We'll discuss how having a support system enhances motivation, provides encouragement, and transforms exercise into a social and enjoyable experience.

The Dance of Practicality: Integrating Exercise into Daily Life

In the midst of busy schedules, the dance of exercise often faces the challenge of practicality. However, with a bit of creativity and strategic planning, you can seamlessly integrate movement into your daily life. Let's explore practical tips to make exercise an integral part of your routine.

Short Bursts of Activity: The Dance of Efficiency

Who says exercise has to be an hour-long commitment? Short bursts of activity, such as taking the stairs, doing quick home workouts, or stretching during breaks, become the dance of efficiency. We'll share practical ways to incorporate micro-workouts into your day, ensuring that movement becomes a natural and efficient part of your routine.

Incorporating Movement into Daily Tasks: The Dance of Integration

Turn daily tasks into a dance of integration by incorporating movement. Whether it's walking or cycling to work, doing squats while brushing your teeth, or dancing while cooking, we'll explore how to infuse movement into your everyday activities. This dance of integration not only adds to your daily exercise but also makes it more enjoyable.

Scheduling Exercise: The Dance of Prioritization

Scheduling exercise is the dance of prioritization that ensures movement receives its dedicated space in your calendar. We'll discuss the importance of treating exercise as a non-negotiable appointment, prioritizing your well-being, and creating a consistent routine.

Personalizing Your Dance: Crafting a Tailored Exercise Plan

Now, let's craft a personalized exercise plan – a dance routine that aligns with your goals, preferences, and lifestyle. This plan is not a rigid set of rules but a flexible guide, allowing you to tailor your dance of exercise to suit your unique rhythm.

Assessing Your Fitness Level: The Dance of Self-Discovery

Begin by assessing your current fitness level. Consider factors such as your health status, any existing medical conditions, and your familiarity with different forms of exercise. This dance of self-discovery forms the foundation for crafting a plan that is both challenging and realistic.

Defining Your Goals: The Dance of Aspiration

What are your dance aspirations? Whether it's improving cardiovascular health, building strength, enhancing flexibility, or simply enjoying the joy of movement, define your goals clearly. This dance of aspiration becomes the guiding star for your personalized exercise plan.

Choosing Your Dance Styles: The Dance of Variety

Select dance styles that resonate with you. If you love the exhilaration of cardio, consider activities like running, cycling, or dancing. If strength and resilience are your dance partners, incorporate weightlifting or bodyweight exercises. This dance of variety ensures that your routine remains engaging and enjoyable.

Creating a Weekly Schedule: The Dance of Consistency

Craft a weekly schedule that incorporates different forms of exercise. This dance of consistency involves setting aside dedicated time for cardio, strength training, flexibility, and mind-body practices. We'll guide you in creating a well-rounded routine that addresses all facets of physical fitness.

Gradual Progression: The Dance of Growth

The dance of growth involves gradual progression. Start at a pace that feels comfortable, gradually increasing the intensity and duration of your workouts. This dance of growth not only prevents injury but also ensures that your body adapts to the demands of your exercise routine.

Celebrating Your Dance: Acknowledging Milestones and Progress

As you embark on your dance of exercise, take moments to celebrate your milestones and progress. Whether it's reaching a fitness goal, mastering a new dance move, or simply staying consistent with your routine, every step is a victory. The dance of celebration adds a layer of joy to your journey, reinforcing the positive impact of exercise on your well-being.

Setting Milestone Celebrations: The Dance of Recognition

Define milestones along your journey and celebrate them. Whether it's completing a certain number of workouts, running a specific distance, or achieving a fitness level, this dance of recognition acknowledges your dedication and achievements.

Tracking Progress: The Dance of Reflection

Keep a record of your progress, noting improvements in strength, endurance, flexibility, and mood. This dance of reflection serves as a motivating reminder of how far you've come. Use a fitness journal, tracking apps, or visual cues to witness the positive changes your dance of exercise brings.

Sharing Your Achievements: The Dance of Community

Share your achievements with your support system, whether it's friends, family, or your accountability partners. This dance of community not only amplifies the joy of your victories but also creates a network of encouragement. Your successes become an inspiration for others on their dance of well-being.

The Ongoing Dance of Exercise: A Lifelong Commitment

As we conclude our exploration of Exercise and Movement, remember that this is not a short-lived performance but a lifelong dance. Your relationship with movement is a dynamic, evolving journey that adapts and grows with you. The chapters ahead will unravel the impact of sleep, nutrition, and mindfulness on your overall well-being, creating a holistic tapestry for your Mind-Body Reset journey.

Until then, dance to the rhythm of your heart, let the beats of your footsteps resonate with joy, and relish the energy that comes from the dance of exercise. You are not just moving; you are celebrating the symphony of your well-being. So, let the dance continue!

CHAPTER 8. WEEK BY WEEK PROGRAM: YOUR GUIDED DANCE OF TRANSFORMATION

As we waltz into This Chapter, envision this as the heart of our program – the Week-by-Week Guide to your transformative journey. Picture it as your personal dance instructor, leading you through the intricacies of breaking free from food addiction, nurturing emotional intelligence, embracing exercise, and crafting a well-balanced, mindful life. So, tighten your shoelaces, adjust your crown, and let's dive into the week-by-week program designed to sculpt the masterpiece that is your renewed self.

Week 1-2: Setting the Stage for Awareness and Reflection

The first steps in any dance are crucial, and your Mind-Body Reset journey is no exception. During these initial weeks, our focus is on setting the stage for self-awareness and reflection – the cornerstones of transformative change.

Daily Journaling and Self-Reflection

- Embrace the dance of self-awareness through daily journaling. Jot down your thoughts, emotions, and experiences.
- Reflect on your relationship with food, identifying patterns and triggers.
- Begin noticing moments of mindless eating or emotional indulgence without judgment.

Introduction to Mindful Eating Practices

- Engage in mindful eating exercises, savoring each bite consciously.
- Explore the sensations, flavors, and textures of your meals without distractions.
- Observe your body's hunger and fullness cues, fostering a mindful connection with nourishment.

Goal-Setting for Awareness

- Set realistic goals for increasing awareness of your eating habits.
- Define achievable targets, such as incorporating mindful eating practices into one meal per day.
- Celebrate small victories, acknowledging moments of heightened awareness.

Week 3-4: Breaking Unhealthy Habits and Cravings

With a foundation of awareness in place, it's time to shift our focus to breaking free from unhealthy habits and unraveling the mystery of cravings. This phase involves introducing strategies to overcome the allure of familiar, but often detrimental, eating patterns.

Identifying Cravings and Triggers

- Delve deeper into understanding your cravings and their triggers.
- Utilize the self-reflection tools introduced in Week 1-2 to identify emotional and situational cues.

- Begin creating a list of alternative activities to engage in when cravings arise.

Mindful Eating as a Cravings Tool

- Strengthen your mindful eating practices as a shield against mindless cravings.
- When a craving strikes, engage in mindful breathing and conscious awareness to assess its intensity.
- Experiment with substituting unhealthy snacks with mindful, satisfying alternatives.

Positive Habit Introduction

- Begin introducing positive habits as substitutes for unhealthy ones.
- Explore micro-habits related to nutrition, such as incorporating a daily serving of vegetables or opting for whole grains.
- Share your progress with your support system, celebrating the initiation of positive changes.

Week 5-6: Establishing New Habits and Building a Routine

As the dance of breaking old habits gains momentum, it's time to welcome new stars onto the stage – positive habits and routines. These weeks focus on establishing a dance of consistency, introducing micro-habits, and crafting a daily routine that aligns with your evolving goals.

Micro-Habit Integration

- Dive into the world of micro-habits, introducing small, manageable changes into your daily routine.
- Examples include incorporating a short morning stretch, practicing mindful breathing before meals, or opting for a daily walk.

- Gradually increase the complexity of micro-habits as you become more comfortable with the dance of change.

Building a Daily Routine

- Craft a daily routine that accommodates your new habits seamlessly.
- Define morning and evening rituals that anchor your day in positivity.
- Ensure your routine allows space for mindful practices, exercise, and nourishing meals.

Accountability Check-In

- Connect with your accountability partners or support system for a check-in.
- Share your experience with establishing new habits and routines.

- Discuss challenges and celebrate successes together, reinforcing the sense of community.

Week 7-8: Strengthening Support Systems and Community Engagement

As your dance of transformation progresses, these weeks shine a spotlight on the pillars of support that surround you. Strengthening connections with your support system and engaging with a community become integral components of sustaining positive change.

Active Engagement with Your Support System

- Reflect on the impact of your support system on your journey.
- Share your goals, challenges, and victories with your accountability partners.
- Offer support in return, creating a reciprocal dance of encouragement.

Community Participation

- Engage more actively with your chosen community or support group.
- Attend local events, workshops, or virtual meet-ups related to nutrition and well-being.
- Contribute to discussions, share insights, and celebrate collective achievements.

Evaluation of Routines and Adjustments

- Evaluate the effectiveness of your daily routines and habits.
- Identify areas that require adjustments or improvements.
- Make necessary changes to ensure that your routine remains a dynamic and supportive dance.

Week 9-10: Culmination of Reflection and Preparation for the Next Phase

As we approach the culmination of the initial phase, these weeks focus on deep reflection, celebrating the progress made, and preparing for the upcoming chapters. It's a time to acknowledge the dance of transformation and the steps taken toward a healthier, more mindful lifestyle.

Reflection on the Journey

- Schedule dedicated moments for reflection on your journey.
- Celebrate the milestones achieved and the positive changes in your relationship with food.
- Express gratitude for the support system and community that have been integral to your dance.

Reassessment of Goals

- Reassess your initial goals in light of the progress made.
- Consider adjusting or expanding goals based on your evolving aspirations.
- Set intentions for the upcoming weeks, aligning them with the themes of emotional intelligence, exercise, and holistic well-being.

- Extend the principles of mindful eating to mindful living.
- Explore incorporating mindfulness into other aspects of your daily life, such as work, relationships, and leisure.
- Begin cultivating a holistic approach to well-being, acknowledging the interconnectedness of mind, body, and spirit.

Transition to Emotional Intelligence and Coping Strategies: Weeks 11-12

As we transition to the next chapters of the Mind-Body Reset journey, the focus shifts towards emotional intelligence and coping strategies. These weeks provide a bridge between the foundational phase and the exploration of the emotional landscape, guiding you toward a deeper understanding of your feelings and their impact on overall well-being.

Introduction to Emotional Intelligence Practices

- Begin exploring practices that enhance emotional intelligence.
- Engage in guided exercises that foster self-awareness and emotional regulation.
- Delve into the dance of empathy, practicing active listening and cultivating compassion.

Coping Strategy Toolbox Expansion

- Expand your coping strategy toolbox to include practices for emotional well-being.
- Experiment with mindfulness and meditation as coping mechanisms.
- Explore creative expression, physical activity, and positive affirmations as tools for navigating emotions.

Week-by-Week Emotional Resilience Building

- Adopt a week-by-week approach to building emotional resilience.
- Explore concepts such as acceptance, adaptability, and learning from setbacks.
- Begin integrating stress management techniques into your daily routine.

Personalized Exercise Plan Implementation: Weeks 13-14

With emotional intelligence and coping strategies as your companions, it's time to reintroduce the dance of exercise into your routine. Weeks 13-14 are dedicated to the personalized implementation of your exercise plan, ensuring that movement becomes an integral part of your holistic well-being.

Revisit Your Personalized Exercise Plan

- Review and fine-tune your personalized exercise plan crafted earlier in the program.
- Assess your fitness goals, preferences, and any adjustments needed.

- Reconnect with the joy of movement and its role in enhancing your physical and mental well-being.

Gradual Integration of Exercise

- Gradually integrate your chosen forms of exercise into your routine.
- Begin with manageable durations and intensities, allowing your body to adapt.
- Embrace the dance of progression, celebrating each step toward enhanced fitness.

Accountability Through Movement

- Share your renewed commitment to exercise with your support system.
- Encourage accountability by scheduling joint workouts or sharing exercise goals.
- Celebrate the shared victories of the dance of movement, fostering a collective sense of well-being.

Ongoing Reflection and Celebration: Weeks 15-16

As we approach the midpoint of the Mind-Body Reset program, Weeks 15-16 emphasize ongoing reflection, celebration of achievements, and preparation for the chapters ahead. It's a time to acknowledge the resilience cultivated, the habits formed, and the transformative dance that continues to unfold.

Midpoint Reflection

- Take a comprehensive look at your journey so far, from breaking free from food addiction to embracing exercise.
- Reflect on the integration of emotional intelligence and coping strategies into your daily life.
- Acknowledge the interconnected dance of mind, body, and emotions.

Celebration of Milestones

- Celebrate the milestones reached, whether they be in nutrition, exercise, or emotional well-being.
- Host a personal celebration or share achievements with your support system.
- Recognize the impact of consistent effort on your evolving sense of self.

Mindful Living Check-In
- Conduct a mindful living check-in, assessing how mindfulness has permeated different facets of your life.
- Explore opportunities for further integration of mindful practices into your routine.
- Cultivate gratitude for the transformative dance you've embraced and the positive shifts experienced.

Looking Ahead: Weeks 17-30

As we step into the second half of the program, Weeks 17-30 unfold a tapestry of exploration, deepening your understanding of sleep, nutrition, and the holistic dance of well-being. Each week is dedicated to a specific theme, providing in-depth insights and actionable steps for continued growth.

Exploration of Sleep: Weeks 17-20

- Dive into the dance of sleep, exploring its profound impact on physical and mental well-being.
- Establish a consistent sleep routine, incorporating relaxation practices before bedtime.
- Explore strategies for improving sleep quality and addressing common sleep challenges.

Nutrition and Nourishment: Weeks 21-24

- Shift the spotlight to the dance of nutrition, examining the role of food as fuel for your well-being.

- Explore balanced meal planning, incorporating a variety of nutrient-dense foods.
- Learn about mindful eating practices that enhance your relationship with food and support overall health.

Holistic Well-Being: Weeks 25-30

- Embrace the dance of holistic well-being, weaving together the threads of nutrition, exercise, sleep, and emotional intelligence.
- Explore the interconnected nature of these elements and how they contribute to a balanced, harmonious life.
- Craft a personalized well-being plan that aligns with your values and aspirations.

Final Reflection and Integration: Weeks 31-32

As the Mind-Body Reset program draws to a close, Weeks 31-32 provide a space for final reflection, integration of learnings, and preparation for the continued dance of self-discovery. It's a time to celebrate the transformative journey and lay the foundation for an ongoing dance of well-being.

Comprehensive Program Reflection

- Reflect on the holistic journey encompassing food addiction, emotional intelligence, exercise, sleep, and nutrition.
- Acknowledge the growth, resilience, and positive changes experienced.
- Celebrate the dance of transformation as a continuous, evolving process.

Integration of Learnings into Daily Life

- Integrate the learnings from each chapter into your daily life.
- Ensure that the habits formed, insights gained, and skills developed become integral components of your ongoing dance of well-being.

- Craft a post-program plan for sustaining the positive changes and nurturing continued growth.

Personalized Well-Being Commitment

- Create a personalized well-being commitment that serves as a guiding compass beyond the program.
- Outline the practices, habits, and mindset you will carry forward in your ongoing dance of well-being.
- Share your commitment with your support system, reinforcing accountability and collective celebration.

Ongoing Dance of Well-Being: Beyond the Program

As the formal program concludes, remember that your dance of well-being is an ongoing journey. Beyond Week 32, continue to explore, adapt, and embrace the evolving dance of your life. Whether it's deepening your emotional intelligence, refining your exercise routine, or discovering new facets of well-being, the dance continues.

Monthly Well-Being Check-Ins

- Schedule monthly check-ins to reflect on your ongoing well-being journey.
- Celebrate achievements, reassess goals, and make adjustments as needed.
- Use these check-ins as an opportunity for ongoing self-discovery and growth.

Community Engagement and Support

- Stay connected with your support system and community.
- Share your ongoing experiences, challenges, and victories.
- Continue to be a source of support for others on their well-being journeys.

Mindful Living as a Lifelong Practice

- Embrace mindful living as a lifelong practice.

- Integrate mindfulness into various aspects of your life, fostering a sense of presence and intention.
- Explore new dimensions of mindfulness, such as mindfulness in relationships and mindful decision-making.

Ongoing Exploration of Well-Being Elements

- Continue to explore the elements of well-being introduced during the program.
- Deepen your understanding of the dance of sleep, nutrition, exercise, and emotional intelligence.
- Be open to discovering new practices and insights that contribute to your ongoing dance of holistic well-being.

Final Words: Your Dance, Your Masterpiece

As we conclude this guided journey through the Mind-Body Reset program, remember that the dance is uniquely yours. You are the choreographer, the dancer, and the audience of your own masterpiece. Each step, each choice, and each moment of self-discovery contributes to the beauty of your ongoing dance.

Celebrate the resilience within you, the growth you've cultivated, and the vibrant tapestry of well-being you continue to weave. The Mind-Body Reset is not a destination but a dance, a lifelong exploration of the intricate and harmonious movements that shape the symphony of your well-being. As you step beyond the formal structure of the program, carry the spirit of curiosity, adaptability, and self-compassion into the ongoing dance of your life.

Chapter 9. Maintaining Progress and Long Term Success: Sustaining the Dance of Well-Being

Hello, seasoned dancers of the Mind-Body Reset! As we step into Chapter 9, envision this as the encore of your transformative journey – a guide to maintaining the rhythm, sustaining the dance, and ensuring that the symphony of your well-being continues to play harmoniously. The spotlight is on maintaining progress and achieving long-term success, making this chapter a crucial finale to the structured program. So, grab your metaphorical dance shoes, let the music of wisdom play, and let's explore the keys to sustaining the vibrant dance of your well-being.

The Dance of Consistency: Nurturing Habits for a Lifetime

The Power of Consistency

- Recall the magic of the early weeks, where habits were formed and routines were established.

- The dance of consistency is a lifelong partner in maintaining progress.
- Consistency is not about perfection but about showing up and engaging in positive habits regularly.

Habitual Refinement and Evolution

- Embrace the dance of refinement and evolution.
- Periodically assess your habits and routines, making adjustments as needed.
- Allow your dance to evolve alongside your changing goals, priorities, and aspirations.

The Micro-Habit Symphony

- Micro-habits introduced during the program become the sweet notes in the ongoing symphony.
- Continue to explore and integrate new micro-habits that align with your well-being goals.

- These small, intentional actions collectively shape the dance of your daily life.

Sustaining Mindful Eating Practices: A Nourishing Ballet

Mindful Eating as a Lifelong Ritual

- Reflect on the journey of mindful eating and its impact on your relationship with food.
- Ensure that mindful eating remains a daily ritual, even beyond the formal program.
- The dance of mindful eating fosters a profound connection between your body and the nourishment it receives.

Mindful Decision-Making in Food Choices

- Apply mindfulness to food choices in various settings, including social gatherings and restaurants.

- Make conscious decisions that align with your well-being goals.
- The dance of mindful decision-making extends the principles of awareness to every dining experience.

Occasional Indulgences and Moderation

- Acknowledge the place of occasional indulgences in the dance of a balanced life.
- Practice moderation and mindfulness during special occasions.
- The ability to enjoy treats without guilt is a skill honed in the ongoing dance of mindful living.

The Dynamic Dance of Emotional Intelligence

Continuous Growth in Emotional Intelligence

- View emotional intelligence as a dynamic dance of continuous growth.

- Engage in ongoing practices that enhance self-awareness, self-regulation, and empathy.
- Emotional intelligence is not a destination but a journey of deepening understanding.

Adapting Coping Strategies to Life's Changes

- Life is an ever-changing dance, and your coping strategies must adapt.
- Explore new coping mechanisms that align with the challenges and joys life presents.
- The dance of emotional resilience involves being flexible in the face of change.

Integrating Emotional Intelligence into Relationships

- Extend the principles of emotional intelligence to your relationships.
- Foster open communication, active listening, and empathetic understanding.

- The dance of emotional intelligence creates harmonious connections in all aspects of your life.

The Eternal Dance of Exercise and Movement

Diverse Movement for Lifelong Vitality

- Embrace the diversity of movement to ensure the dance remains vibrant.
- Explore different forms of exercise, adjusting based on your interests and body's needs.
- Lifelong vitality is achieved through a dance that adapts and evolves.

Joyful Movement Beyond Formal Exercise

- Let movement extend beyond structured workouts.
- Engage in activities that bring joy, whether it's dancing in your living room, hiking in nature, or playing a sport.

- The dance of well-being includes a joyful celebration of movement in all its forms.

Social Exercise: A Communal Dance
- Cultivate the joy of social exercise.
- Join classes, clubs, or sports teams to make movement a communal dance.
- The support of a community adds a dynamic and enriching layer to the ongoing dance of physical well-being.

Sleep: The Serenade of Restful Nights

Prioritizing Sleep as a Non-Negotiable
- Reaffirm the importance of sleep as a non-negotiable component of well-being.
- Protect your sleep routine as fiercely as you would any other vital aspect of your health.
- The dance of well-being flourishes in the serenade of restful nights.

Adapting Sleep Practices to Life Changes

- Life's dance may introduce changes in routines, schedules, or responsibilities.
- Adapt your sleep practices to align with these changes, ensuring a consistent and restorative rhythm.
- The dance of sleep is a flexible waltz that harmonizes with the seasons of life.

Quality Over Quantity: The Essence of Sleep

- Focus on the quality of sleep, prioritizing restful and rejuvenating slumber.
- Create an environment conducive to sleep, with attention to darkness, comfort, and relaxation.
- The dance of well-being is elevated when each night becomes a nourishing lullaby for the body and mind.

Nutritional Harmony: Crafting a Sustained Culinary Dance

Balanced Nutrition as a Lifelong Dance

- Nutritional harmony is an ongoing dance of balanced choices.

- Continue to explore a variety of nutrient-dense foods, embracing the richness of culinary diversity.
- The dance of nutrition is a celebration of nourishment, health, and pleasure.

Mindful Eating as a Guiding Principle

- Let mindful eating guide your culinary dance.
- Savor each bite, listen to your body's cues, and appreciate the flavors and textures of your meals.
- The dance of mindful eating transforms each meal into a mindful, intentional experience.

Adventurous Eating: Exploring New Horizons

- Infuse an adventurous spirit into your nutritional dance.

- Explore new recipes, cuisines, and cooking techniques to keep the dance exciting.
- The journey of well-being is not just about sustenance but a dance of culinary exploration.

Holistic Well-Being: The Symphony of Integration

Interconnected Well-Being Components

- View the elements of well-being as interconnected threads in a vibrant tapestry.
- Ensure each component – nutrition, exercise, sleep, and emotional intelligence – contributes harmoniously to the dance.
- The symphony of well-being is a collective expression of a life lived in balance.

Ongoing Mindful Living Practices

- Extend the principles of mindful living beyond the initial program.
- Let mindfulness permeate your work, relationships, and leisure.
- The dance of well-being unfolds as you navigate life with intention, presence, and gratitude.

Community and Support as Pillars of Strength

- Maintain strong connections with your support system and community.
- Share your ongoing experiences, challenges, and triumphs.
- The dance of well-being is enriched when it's a shared celebration with those who support and inspire you.

Monthly Reflection: A Rhythmic Check-In

Monthly Well-Being Audits Revisited

- Revisit the practice of monthly well-being audits.
- Reflect on the balance of different elements in your well-being dance.
- Use these regular check-ins as compass points for maintaining the rhythm of your ongoing dance.

Continuous Goal Setting and Celebration

- Continue setting and reassessing your well-being goals.
- Celebrate both small and significant milestones, reinforcing the dance of progress.
- The journey of well-being is not a linear path but a dance of continuous growth and self-discovery.

The Role of Mindfulness in the Lifelong Dance

Mindfulness as the Heartbeat of Well-Being

- Acknowledge mindfulness as the heartbeat of your well-being dance.
- Cultivate mindfulness in every aspect of your life, from daily routines to significant decisions.
- The dance of well-being is elevated when it's guided by a mindful, intentional presence.

Mindful Decision-Making in Life Choices

- Extend mindfulness to life choices, both big and small.
- Approach decisions with a clear mind, considering the alignment with your values and well-being goals.
- The dance of well-being is a conscious journey where each step is a mindful choice.

Gratitude and Reflection: The Dance of Acknowledgment

Gratitude as a Guiding Light

- Infuse your ongoing dance with the spirit of gratitude.
- Regularly express appreciation for the elements of well-being, supportive relationships, and the beauty of life.
- The dance of well-being is a celebration of the blessings and abundance that surround you.

Reflection as a Source of Growth
- Continue the practice of reflection, acknowledging the growth and lessons of your journey.
- The dance of well-being thrives when each step is an opportunity for learning and self-discovery.
- Reflection becomes a compass that guides your ongoing dance toward greater depth and authenticity.

Evolving Goals: A Dance of Aspiration

Reassessment and Expansion of Goals

- Periodically reassess your well-being goals, expanding them based on your evolving aspirations.
- The dance of well-being is a dynamic journey, and your goals should reflect the ever-unfolding nature of your path.
- Embrace new challenges and aspirations as integral components of your ongoing dance.

Incorporating Well-Being into Life Milestones

- Integrate well-being into life milestones, whether they be personal, professional, or relational.
- The dance of well-being is not separate from the fabric of your life but an integral part of the grand tapestry of your existence.
- Celebrate achievements with the awareness that well-being is not a destination but an ongoing dance.

The Lifelong Dance of Well-Being: A Final Overture

As we conclude our exploration of maintaining progress and achieving long-term success, remember that the dance of well-being is not a fleeting performance but a lifelong journey. It's an ongoing symphony where each element – nutrition, exercise, sleep, emotional intelligence, and mindful living – contributes to the harmonious composition of your life.

As you step into the encore of your well-being dance, embrace the principles, habits, and wisdom gained during the program. Let them be the guiding notes in the ongoing composition of your life. The Mind-Body Reset has provided a foundation, but the dance is yours to choreograph.

Ongoing Community Engagement: Dance Partners for Life

Community as a Supportive Ensemble

- Maintain strong connections with your support system and community.
- Engage in regular check-ins, sharing experiences and offering encouragement.

- The dance of well-being is richer and more joyful when it's a shared celebration.

Collective Wisdom and Inspiration

- Draw upon the collective wisdom of your community for ongoing inspiration.
- Share your insights and learn from the experiences of others.
- The dance of well-being is an ever-evolving dialogue, with each participant contributing to the collective wisdom.

The Mind-Body Reset Legacy: A Gift to Future Generations

Sharing Your Journey: A Guiding Light

- Consider sharing your well-being journey as a source of inspiration for others.
- Your experiences, challenges, and triumphs can serve as a guiding light for

those embarking on their own dance of well-being.

- The legacy of the Mind-Body Reset extends beyond personal transformation to become a gift to future generations.

Passing on the Wisdom of Well-Being

- If you have the opportunity, pass on the wisdom of well-being to those around you.
- Whether it's friends, family, or colleagues, share the principles of mindful living, emotional intelligence, and holistic well-being.
- The dance of well-being becomes a ripple effect, touching the lives of those you inspire.

Final Reflection: The Ongoing Overture

As we reach the final notes of this chapter, take a moment for reflection. Consider the progress you've made, the lessons you've learned, and the ongoing dance that lies ahead. The Mind-Body Reset program has equipped you with tools, insights, and a roadmap for well-being, but the dance is yours to lead.

In the grand ballroom of life, may your dance be filled with vitality, joy, and a deep sense of purpose. Each step is a brushstroke on the canvas of your existence, creating a masterpiece of well-being. As the curtain falls on this chapter, the overture of your lifelong well-being dance continues.

Dance on, resilient soul, dance on!

Conclusion: A Flourishing Final to Your Mind-Body Reset Journey

As you stand at the brink of the final chapter, envision it as not just the conclusion of a book but the flourishing finale to a transformative journey – your Mind-Body Reset journey. You've traversed the pages, embraced the challenges, and danced through the rhythms of breaking free from food addiction. Now, let's take a moment to revel in the collective triumphs, reflect on the tapestry of growth woven over the past 30 days, and set the stage for the continued dance of well-being in your life.

Reflecting on Your Journey: Celebrating Victories Big and Small

Acknowledging Progress: A Dance of Triumphs

- Pause and acknowledge the milestones you've achieved.
- Whether it's a newfound awareness of emotional triggers, the establishment of nourishing eating habits, or the joy of

movement reintegrated into your routine, celebrate each victory with the gusto it deserves.

- Your journey is a testament to resilience, determination, and the transformative power of intentional choices.

The Dance of Resilience: Triumph Over Challenges

- Reflect on the challenges you encountered and overcame.
- The dance of resilience is a recurring theme in your story – from navigating cravings to facing emotional hurdles.
- Every challenge met and conquered has contributed to the strength and resilience you now carry forward.

The Art of Mindful Living: A Canvas of Well-Being

- Consider how mindfulness has become a brushstroke in the canvas of your daily life.

- The mindful living practices introduced in the program are now part of your repertoire, guiding your decisions, actions, and interactions.
- The art of mindful living is not just a tool but a masterpiece in the ongoing creation of your well-being.

The Holistic Tapestry: Weaving Nutrition, Exercise, and Emotional Resilience

Nutrition: From Fuel to Harmony

- Revisit the nutritional dance you've engaged in over the past 30 days.
- From mindful eating to crafting balanced meals, you've transformed the act of nourishment into a harmonious dance.
- Nutrition is no longer just about fuel; it's an integral part of your holistic well-being.

Exercise: From Routine to Joyful Movement

- Think about how exercise has evolved from a routine to a joyful dance.

- Whether it's a solo workout, a community class, or a nature hike, movement has become an expression of joy and vitality.
- The dance of exercise is a celebration of the incredible capabilities of your body.

Emotional Resilience: The Heartbeat of Well-Being

- Consider the strides you've made in understanding and managing your emotions.
- The emotional resilience dance involves acknowledging, processing, and responding to emotions in a healthy way.
- Emotional intelligence is not just a skill; it's the heartbeat of your well-being journey.

Personal Transformation: Embracing a New Chapter

Breaking Free from Food Addiction: A Liberating Dance

- Reflect on the freedom you've cultivated from food addiction.

- The dance of liberation involves releasing the chains that bound you to unhealthy eating patterns.
- You've taken the reins of your relationship with food, shaping it into a source of nourishment rather than a coping mechanism.

A Renewed Sense of Self: The Dance of Discovery

- Take a moment to connect with the evolving sense of self.
- The dance of self-discovery is ongoing, and each step has revealed new facets of your strengths, preferences, and aspirations.
- Embrace the ever-unfolding journey of becoming the best version of yourself.

The Mind-Body Connection: A Symbiotic Dance

- Consider the harmonious connection you've fostered between mind and body.

- The mind-body dance is a symbiotic relationship where each element influences and supports the other.
- Your journey exemplifies the transformative power of aligning mental and physical well-being.

The Week-by-Week Unveiling: A Guided Odyssey

The Guided Journey: From Weeks 1 to 32

- Think back to the structured weeks that unfolded the program.
- Each week brought new insights, challenges, and triumphs, guiding you through the intricacies of breaking free from food addiction.
- The week-by-week approach was a roadmap, and you've successfully navigated its twists and turns.

Community and Support: A Dance of Connection

- Reflect on the role of community and support in your journey.
- Whether through shared experiences, encouragement, or accountability, your dance has been enriched by the support system around you.
- The community is not just a backdrop but an integral part of your well-being narrative.

Mindful Living Beyond the Program: A Lifelong Dance

- Consider how mindful living practices have transcended the program structure.
- Mindfulness is not a checkbox but a continuous dance, shaping your daily experiences and interactions.
- The dance of mindfulness is a lifelong journey of presence, intention, and gratitude.

Looking Ahead: A Dance of Possibilities

Beyond Week 32: Your Ongoing Well-Being Dance

- As you stand on the threshold of the final chapter, envision the chapters yet to be written.
- Your well-being dance is not confined to the structured program; it's an ongoing exploration of possibilities.
- Each step forward is a note in the symphony of your continued well-being.

Monthly Check-Ins: A Rhythmic Pulse

- Embrace the practice of monthly well-being check-ins.
- These rhythmic pulses provide moments of reflection, celebration, and course correction in the ongoing dance of your life.
- Monthly check-ins are not just a tool but a celebration of your commitment to well-being.

The Ever-Unfolding Dance: A Lifelong Symphony

- Consider your well-being journey as an ever-unfolding dance.
- There is no final destination; rather, it's a continuous exploration of self, growth, and joyful living.
- The dance of well-being is a lifelong symphony, and you are both the composer and the conductor.

Final Words: Your Ongoing Overture

As we draw the curtain on the Mind-Body Reset journey, let these final words resonate in your heart: Your dance is uniquely yours, and the music of well-being is composed by your intentional choices, resilience, and commitment to growth. As the conductor of your ongoing overture, continue to dance with joy, authenticity, and a deep sense of purpose.

May the notes of well-being reverberate in every aspect of your life – in your relationships, your work, and your self-care. Dance on, resilient soul, dance on! The Mind-Body Reset may be concluding, but your well-being journey is an ever-unfolding dance of possibility and potential.

With heartfelt congratulations on completing the Mind-Body Reset program, here's to the vibrant dance of your continued well-being.

"As you step into the next chapter of your life, may each mindful choice be a brushstroke in the vibrant canvas of your well-being, and may your journey beyond these pages continue to dance with the rhythms of freedom, self-love, and lasting transformation."

Milton Keynes UK
Ingram Content Group UK Ltd.
UKHW022035301123
433552UK00015B/504